Nourish to Flourish

A Comprehensive Guide to Optimal Health

By

Ron N. Miner

Table of contents

Conclusion

INTRODUCTION

Sparking Your Wellness Adventure

Salutations, compatriot, as we set out on the profound journey contained in the pages of **Nourish to Flourish: A Comprehensive Guide to Optimal Health.** This book is your compass, pointing you in the direction of a brighter future when health is a voyage rather than a far-off beach.

Setting Out on an Expedition to Radiant Health: An Underpinning to Well-Being

You may wonder why you should go on this quest. The plethora of benefits in store for you holds the solution. These chapters will reveal the transformational power of food and open your eyes to a wealth of benefits that go well beyond traditional conceptions of health.

My drive as an author comes from a love of discovering the mysteries that lie beneath the food that we eat. The profound research I did into the remarkable therapeutic qualities of particular foods gave rise to this book. Imagine this as a cookbook, a recipe book that has been painstakingly created to arm you with the knowledge to fight diseases that may be lurking inside of you as well as to say goodbye to extra fat and take on the obstacles that obesity presents.

As varied as the nutrients your body will receive, so too are the benefits you stand to receive. This book is your friend in learning how to prepare meals that are powerful healers as well as palate tantalizers. It's a road map for losing weight and illnesses that sap your energy levels.

Therefore, consider this introduction to be a call to action—an invitation to begin your journey toward wellness and reap the rewards that lie ahead. No matter how many pages you flip, you're not just learning; you're learning how to thrive—a brilliant metamorphosis that starts on the inside and is driven by the profound relationship between what you eat and the robust health you deserve.

Chapter one

Weaving Well-Being Through Nutritional Tapestry

This chapter provides access to a thorough understanding of optimal health within the broad context of well-being. It is an investigation into the complex web of choices our body nutrition choices create. Imagine this chapter as a rich continuation that goes deeper into the fabric of wellbeing, carrying on the adventure that was started in the introduction.

A Culinary Odyssey Revealed: A Follow-Up to the Introduction

When the curtain rises on the nutritional stage, eating becomes a gastronomic voyage, a symphony of flavours, textures, and nutrients that can prolong life. The nutritional tapestry is a live, breathing organism that is woven with each mouthful, a canvas on which your bright health is revealed. It is not merely a metaphor.

Deciphering the Code of a Bright Life: Culinary Alchemy Expounded

To uncover the first mystery, let's take off the layers of this tapestry: Sulforaphane, a substance with strong anti-inflammatory and antioxidant qualities, is found in broccoli, the unsung hero of the vegetable kingdom. Consider every floret not only as a garnish but also as a barrier against cellular harm.

After that, travel to the blueberry world. These little balls of goodness have a hidden cache of antioxidants that help protect against oxidative stress and improve cognitive function. Your daily bowl of oats becomes a source of beta-glucans, which promote heart health and regulate cholesterol levels, in addition to being a filling breakfast.

Garlic is another example of culinary alchemy; it is not only a flavor enhancer but also a natural antibacterial that strengthens your immune system. Salmon and other fatty fish provide omega-3 fatty acids that improve mental health and cognitive function in addition to being a delicious treat for the brain.

Extra Culinary Treasures: The Seven Secrets of Nature

1. Curcuma: The curcumin-rich golden spice has anti-inflammatory and antioxidant qualities that promote immunological system and joint health.

2. Verdant: Beyond just being a leafy green, it also contains high levels of iron, magnesium, and vitamin K, all of which support healthy bones and general vigor.

3. Avocado: It aids in nutrition absorption and heart health because it is high in monounsaturated fats.

4. Nuts: Omega-3 fatty acids, which improve cognitive function and reduce inflammation, can be found in these brain-shaped nuts.

5. Chia Seeds: Rich in fiber and omega-3 fatty acids, they facilitate better digestion and support heart health.

6. Sweet Potatoes: Rich in vitamins A and C, they support healthy skin and a strong immune system.

7. Tea Verde: Antioxidants and substances that promote metabolism and general wellbeing are found in this beverage, which has been consumed for centuries.

These seven dietary tips are only a small part of the enormous tapestry of foods that are the secret to vibrant health. Think of this chapter as the compass that will lead you across the rich terrain of optimal health in the upcoming chapters. Each meal will act as a brushstroke, adding to the masterpiece that is your well-being.

Chapter two

Culinary Alchemy: Crafting Healing Plates

Enter the realm of culinary alchemy, where the artistry of creating dishes goes beyond providing nourishment and becomes a healing process intended to infuse taste with meaning and promote overall well being. We will discover how to create flavour profiles that are restorative, comprehend the health benefits of each component, and adopt a diet that nourishes the body and spirit in addition to nourishment in this chapter.

The Secrets of Culinary Alchemy: From Flavour to Whole Health

Culinary alchemy is the union of flavours and purpose that transforms each meal into a symphony of flavour, nourishment, and healing. Your plate is a painting on which every component plays a part in creating a symphony that speaks to your wellbeing, not just a collection of components.

Building Restorative Taste Profiles: A Musical Symphony on Your Plate

1.   Turmeric-Infused   Quinoa Bowl: Turmeric's   anti-inflammatory curcumin both gives the quinoa a toasty golden colour and helps to lower inflammation in the body.

2. Salmon with Ginger and Garlic: In addition to their flavorful appeal, ginger   and   garlic   provide anti-inflammatory   and immune-stiffening qualities that improve general health with every juicy bite.

3. Salad of mango and avocado with chilli-lime dressing: The creamy avocado's healthful fats complement the mango's sweetness, and the chili-lime dressing adds flavour and vitamins C and improves metabolism.

4. Rosemary Roasted SweetPotatoes: Rosemary lends a lovely scent to the sweet potatoes and also contributes antioxidants that improve their vitamin and fibre content.

The Alchemy of Combining Flavours to Get the Most Impact

Think of the skill of pairing as a tactical alliance between tastes and wellness advantages. Often linked to warmth and sweetness, cinnamon improves taste and helps to keep blood sugar levels stable. When combined with cilantro, cumin produces a harmonious blend of earthy and fresh flavours that supports digestion and is a rich source of vital minerals.

Meditative Eating: Appreciating the Symphony

Mindful eating improves the whole experience in addition to its nutritional advantages. Using all of your senses when consuming food helps you develop a more intimate relationship with it and promotes a fuller, more emotional and mental approach to feeding.

Every taste is a note in the music of your well-being, so keep that in mind when you set out to create healing plates. In addition to offering recipes, this chapter encourages you to use your plate as a blank canvas to create a diet that nourishes your body and your soul.

Chapter Three

Nature's Healing Elixirs
Uncovering Superfoods

A journey into the world of nutritional marvels awaits you as common foods become amazing superfoods—Nature's Healing Elixirs. In this chapter, we will take a deeper look at effective cures and the wide range of superfoods that can be both a powerful ally and a source of nourishment on the path to optimal health.

A Search for the Powerful Curatives in the Natural World

Consider this chapter as a treasure hunt, where each superfood reveals a clue that could lead to a powerful cure. We're going to go on a culinary journey that goes beyond the norm, discovering the therapeutic potential concealed in the center of nature, with stops along the way from ancient grains to vivid berries.

Natural Diet and Tastes for Overweight and Obesity: A Nutritional Journey

1. Chia Seeds: These minuscule seeds expand to create a gel-like substance that satisfies hunger. Rich in fiber and heart-healthy omega-3 fatty acids, they help control weight and promote general heart health.

2. Evergreen Tea: Green tea, especially the catechins in it, is a powerful antioxidant in addition to being a calming beverage. These substances might support the body's fat-burning processes by increasing metabolism.

3. Quinoa: Being a complete protein source, quinoa has fiber and vital amino acids, which help with satiety and weight management. It is a fantastic supplement to a balanced diet because of its adaptability.

4. Raspberries, Blueberries, and Strawberries): Berries are a sweet and gratifying method to fulfill cravings because they are high in antioxidants, vitamins, and fiber. Because of their high nutrient density and low calorie content, they are perfect for assisting with weight loss.

5. Avocado: Avocados are high in fiber and minerals, which helps you feel fuller even though they are high in healthy fats. Improved weight management has been linked to avocados' monounsaturated fats.

6. Oats: Oats are high in soluble fiber, which helps you feel fuller and releases energy gradually. They make a nutritious breakfast choice that can help manage hunger all day.

7. Salmon: A fatty fish such as salmon gives a source of high-quality protein in addition to omega-3 fatty acids. These components promote general health and help one feel full.

Developing Taste-Bomb Superfood Recipes: A Gastronomic Journey

1. Chia Seed dessert with Berries Mix chia seeds with almond milk and add a berry mélange on top for a tasty and filling dessert that is high in antioxidants and omega-3 fatty acids.

2. Green Tea Smoothie: - This nutrient-dense smoothie boosts metabolism by blending green tea, spinach, banana, and a small amount of honey. It is refreshing and hydrating.

3. Salmon and Avocado Quinoa Salad: Toss cooked quinoa with flaked salmon and avocado slices to make a hearty salad. For a tasty and filling dinner, drizzle with a mild vinaigrette.

This chapter walks you through incorporating these healing elixirs into your everyday meals while also revealing the best superfoods nature has to offer through a culinary adventure. Remember that achieving optimal health is a journey rather than a goal as you investigate these superfoods; along the way, the tastes of nature will support you as you strive to thrive.

Chapter Four

Gastronomic Medicine:Treating Illnesses With Food

We uncover the profound relationship between our diet and how it affects our health via the study of gastronomic medicine. Let's first discuss the definition of Gastronomic Medicine, its importance, and the fundamentals of Epicurean Solutions before delving into the Epicurean Solutions that promote everyday wellness.

Definition of Gastronomic Medicine: Savouring Healing Possibilities

The practice of using food as a therapeutic tool to prevent, treat, and mitigate different types of illnesses is known as gastronomic medicine. It acknowledges that the foods we select, the method we cook them, and the customs around mealtimes all play a role in both healing and nourishing. It's a holistic approach that recognizes the relationship between flavour, nutrition, and overall health.

A Culinary Prescription for Health: The Significance of Gastronomic Medicine

Gastronomic medicine is important because it can enable people to actively participate in their own health. We can treat a variety of illnesses organically by knowing the therapeutic qualities of various foods and deliberately mixing them. By transforming each meal into a purposeful act of self-care, this method improves both physical health and the entire sense of feeding.

Epicurean Solutions: Alchemy of Food for Well-Being

Epicurean Solutions are carefully designed cures that combine culinary concepts with the goal of health. These are tasty and savoury mixtures made to address particular health issues rather than just pills. To put it simply, Epicurean Solutions stress that healing via food doesn't always need sacrifice, but rather involves a journey of savouring and relishing satisfying meals.

Let's now examine 25 Epicurean Remedies for a variety of illnesses, along with a thorough explanation of how to make each remedy:

1. Drowsiness: Chamomile Tea - Before going to bed, soak some dried chamomile flowers in a cup of hot water.

Give it 5-7 minutes to infuse. If preferred, add honey.

2. Article Pain: Golden Milk with Turmeric: Add honey, turmeric, and a dash of black pepper to warm milk of your choice. To make a calming golden milk, thoroughly stir.

3. Integumentary Disorders: Ginger Infusion

Fresh ginger should be sliced and steeped in boiling water. Garnish with a little honey and lemon, if desired. Prior to drinking, strain.

4. Common Cold: Chicken Soup: Use herbs, spices, and veggies to gently simmer chicken to make a filling and healthy soup.

5. Depression: Rich Chocolate-Berry Smoothie - Make a tasty smoothie with dark chocolate, berries, yoghourt, and banana to help reduce anxiety.

6. Garlic Roasted Salmon: for High Blood Pressure - Marinate fish with herbs, olive oil, and minced garlic. Cook thoroughly by roasting or grilling.

7. Kale and Walnut Salad: Osteoporosis, Mix kale, walnuts, and a lemon vinaigrette to create a nutrient-rich salad that promotes bone health.

8. Acne: Green Tea Face Mask: For possible skin-soothing benefits, combine green tea leaves with honey and use as a face mask.

9. Headaches: Peppermint Infused Water Pour cold water over fresh peppermint leaves to create a relaxing beverage.

10. Almond and Banana Smoothie Bowl: for stress
Make a smoothie with almonds, banana, and yoghourt. For a bowl that relieves stress, top with oats and fresh fruits.

11. Hair Elixir from Local Honey: For Allergies. Combine one tsp of regional honey with warm water. Regular use may help reduce the symptoms of allergies.

12. Arthritis Pineapplef of Turmeric Smoothie - Blend coconut water, pineapple, and turmeric to make a cool smoothie that may have anti-inflammatory properties.

13. Depression: Lemon-Squeezed Mackerel Mackerel is a high source of omega-3 fatty acids, which are known to boost mental health. Grill it with a squeeze of lemon.

14. Memory Boost: Blueberry Walnut Parfait Arrange yoghourt, walnuts, and blueberries to create a parfait that is full of nutrients and antioxidants that help the brain function.

15. After a night of excess: Hydrate with Coconut Water Sip coconut water to restore electrolytes and hydrate your body.

16. Eczema: Mask with Avocado and Oatmeal
   - To make a calming face mask that can help with eczema symptoms, mash one avocado and combine it with oats.

17. Anaemia: Lentil Spinach Stew - To make a dish high in iron and vitamin C, cook a substantial stew with lentils, spinach, and tomatoes.

18. Infusion of Ginger Tea for Menstrual Cramps, Prepare ginger tea by steeping fresh ginger in boiling water. Add honey if desired for sweetness.

19. Gut Health: Kimchi Quinoa Bowl – Use kimchi to add flavour and gut health to a quinoa bowl with veggies.

20. Cranberry Orange Juice for Bladder Infections: Combine fresh orange juice and unsweetened cranberry juice to make a beverage that may help ward off bladder infections.

21. Hangnails: Almond Oil Moisturizer – To moisturise and avoid hangnails, periodically apply almond oil to your cuticles.

22. Sweetheart: Aloe Vera Drink - Mix aloe vera gel, yoghourt, cucumber, and mint to make a calming smoothie that can help with heartburn.

23. Post-Exercise Tart Cherry Recovery Drink: May Help Reduce Muscle Soreness – Blend coconut water and tart cherry juice to make a post-exercise beverage.

24. Dehydrated Skin: Olive Oil Bath Soak - To relieve and moisturize dry skin, add a couple teaspoons of olive oil to a warm bath.

25. Insulin Resistance: Cinnamon-Spiced Oatmeal –Add a dash of cinnamon to oatmeal to help with blood sugar regulation and perhaps increase insulin sensitivity.

These Epicurean Solutions are invitations to explore the restorative power of food in ways beyond recipes.

Chapter Five

Mindful Taste, Mindful Thought: An Equilibrium Partnership

This chapter takes us into the domain of symbiotic harmony—the dance between the palate and the mind. A voyage into the relationship between food and mental health is offered by "Mindful Palate, Mindful Mind". In addition to learning which foods and flavours are perhaps best avoided for optimal health, this chapter will examine how the decisions we make regarding what to eat can have a significant impact on our mental health.

Uncovering the Linked Universe of Nutrition and Mental Wellness

Imagine the food on your plate as a canvas, with each ingredient adding a different colour to the masterpiece that is your mental health. In "Mindful Palate, Mindful Mind," we explore the science and practice of feeding the mind in addition to the body. Our decisions in the kitchen have an impact on all facets of our lives and are not isolated.

Savours and Foods for a Fulfilled Thought: A Gastronomic Symphony

1. Salmon and mackerel are examples of fatty fish.

These fish, which are high in omega-3 fatty acids, support brain function and may lower the risk of mental health problems.

2. Verdant Vegetables: Kale and Spinach- Rich in vitamins and folate, leafy greens aid maintain brain health and may even stave off cognitive ageing.

3. Nuts and Seeds: Flaxseeds and Walnuts - These seeds and nuts, which are rich in minerals, antioxidants, and omega-3 fatty acids, support brain function in general.

4. Strawberries and blueberries are the berries. Berries contain antioxidants that may help slow down the ageing of the brain and have been related to better cognition.

5. Dark Chocolate - Packed with flavonoids, dark chocolate may improve cognitive function by increasing blood flow to the brain.

6. Turmeric - The component that makes up turmeric, curcumin, has antioxidant and anti-inflammatory properties that may help with brain function.

7. Broccoli - Broccoli supports the general health of the nervous system because it is rich in antioxidants and vitamin K.

Foods and Flavors to Minimise or Steer Clear of for Mental Health

While some meals support mental health, others may hinder the mind's ability to function at its best. Here are some foods and flavours you might want to moderate or stay away from:

1. Too Much Sugar- Consuming too much sugar has been connected to inflammation and may have a detrimental effect on cognitive performance.

2. Foods that have been processed Processed foods, being high in unhealthy

fats and additives, have been linked to mental health problems.

3. Trans Fats – Included in several commercially baked and fried foods, trans fats may be harmful to cognitive function.

4. Artificial Sweeteners – Research points to a possible connection between artificial sweeteners and mental health issues.

The consumption of Highly Processed and Fried Foods may raise one's risk of anxiety and depression.

6. Excessive Alcohol-Alcoholism can have a detrimental effect on mental health, even though moderate consumption can have some health benefits.

Plating an Intentional Meal: A Mindful Approach

The way you approach each meal is just as important to mindful eating as the items on your plate. Take into account these actions:

1. Savour Every Bite: Give your food a real taste and enjoy it thoroughly. Observe the fragrances, tastes, and textures.

2. Exercise Appreciation - Recognize the work that went into getting the food on your plate. Thank you for providing the food.

3. Eat with Awareness: Reduce interruptions during eating. Switch off the screens and concentrate on your meal.

4. Listen to Your Body: – Pay attention to indications that indicate fullness and hunger. When hungry, eat, and when full, stop.

5. Balanced Nutrition: Make an effort to eat a diverse and well-balanced diet that provides a range of nutrients for your body and mind.

As suggested in "Mindful Palate, Mindful Mind," use every meal as an opportunity to nourish your mind as well as your body. Let mindfulness guide your decisions as we explore the interrelated realm of food and mental health, resulting in a beautiful symphony that echoes across all facets of your flourishing well-being.

Chapter Six

The Nourishment Revolution: Lifelong Sustainable Habits

We go out on "The Nourishment Revolution," a journey that goes beyond personal well-being to transform health via deliberate dietary decisions, in this crucial chapter. Along the way, we'll discover sustainable practices that can improve not just our personal lives but also the health of the entire world.

Conscious Nutritional Choices: Revolutionising Health

1. Vegan-Powered Cuisine:

A diet high in fruits, vegetables, legumes, and whole grains that is primarily plant-based should be adopted. Making this decision improves one's own health as well as lessens the impact of food production on the environment.

2. Conscientious Ingestion:

- Eat mindfully by focusing on the nourishment your meal gives, enjoying each bite, and savouring the flavours. This improves digestion and creates a positive relationship between the person and food.

3. Restaurants and Seasonal Food:

- Select seasonal and locally grown goods. This decision guarantees fresher, more nutrient-dense fruit while also boosting the local economy.

4. Diverse Consumption of Nutrients:

Incorporate a range of vibrant fruits and veggies into your meals to aim for a varied spectrum of nutrients. In addition to guaranteeing a wide range of vital vitamins and minerals, this enhances general health.

5. Keeping Macronutrients in Balance:

- Keep an eye on the proportions of the three macronutrients: proteins, lipids, and carbohydrates. A balanced diet promotes optimal body processes and long-term energy levels.

6. Stations of Hydration:

Make water your main beverage and prioritise staying hydrated. Maintaining proper hydration is essential for good health since it promotes healthy digestion, sharp mind, and glowing skin.

7. Control in Balance:

- Make nutritional choices that are moderate. Treats are fine, but only when given in moderation. This strategy promotes a long-lasting and pleasurable connection with eating.

8. Entire Food Intake:

- Pick unprocessed, whole foods instead of heavily processed ones. Whole foods maintain their fibre and natural nutrients, which aid digestion and general health.

9. Conscience in Meal Planning:

- Make careful meal plans that support your dietary objectives. This method cuts down on food waste while also streamlining your dining habits.

10. Culinary Investigation:

- Try out different and novel dishes to make your meals interesting and fulfilling. You are exposed to a greater variety of nutrients as well as expanding your culinary horizons as a result.

The Ripple Effect: From Individual Well-Being to Global Health

The ecosystem is impacted by the ripple effect of conscious dietary decisions that go beyond the individual. We can lessen our ecological footprint, improve the health of the world, and ensure the welfare of future generations by embracing sustainable behaviours. "The Nourishment Revolution" refers to a collective movement that aims to create a world that is more nourished, sustainable, and interconnected, rather than only being about what we eat. It is not only a decision to join this revolution; it is a pledge to live a fulfilling life while promoting the health of our world.

<u>Conclusion</u>

Absorb More Than Just Food

It's not just the end, but also the beginning of a thriving journey enabled by mindful nourishment as we close the book on our all-inclusive guide to optimal health. We'll explore the essence of living well beyond the plate in this last chapter, providing guidance that goes beyond basic nutrition and promotes a whole-person approach to health.

Nourishing Your Flourishing Journey With Empowerment

Developing well is a journey that never ends and goes beyond what's on your plate. It's not merely a destination. It's about choosing a way of living that takes care of your body, mind, and spirit. While you proceed down this path, keep in mind:

1. "Elevate Your Life, Elevate Your Palate": Every aspect of your life is impacted by the decisions you make at the dinner table. Savour the tastes, take pleasure in the textures, and let every meal turn into a celebration of life.

2. Embrace Variety: - Promote variety in your diet by examining a range of nutrients from various meals. In addition to providing nourishment for your body, a diversified diet keeps your culinary adventure interesting.

3. Pay Attention to the Wisdom of Your Body: - Mindful eating enables you to interpret the messages your body sends out about what it needs. Pay attention to the knowledge of your body and respect its signals of hunger, fullness, and satisfaction.

4. Cultivate Mindful Habits: - Practice awareness outside of the dining room. Practice mindful living by realizing how decisions affect your overall wellbeing and how they are connected to one another.

5. Appreciate Development Rather than Excellence:- Your path to flourishing is a process, not a finish line. On this transforming path, acknowledge and appreciate your modest achievements, and practice self-compassion.

Healthy Eating and Healthy Living

Remember that eating healthfully is an important act of self-love and care as you work toward achieving optimal health.

Here are some suggestions for your path to flourishing:

Make entire Foods a Priority: Make sure to select entire, high-nutrient foods that offer a harmonious blend of minerals, vitamins, and antioxidants. These are the fundamental elements of a healthy body.

Remain Hydrated:

Your life's nectar is water. Maintain proper hydration to aid with digestion, mental clarity, and general energy.

Adjust Your Body

Engaging in physical activity is essential when pursuing optimal health. Make movement a part of your everyday routine by engaging in joyful activities.

Recuperate and Rest

A key component of wellbeing is getting enough sleep. Make getting enough sleep a priority so that your body and mind can recover.

Promote Emotional Wellbeing

Nurture your emotional health with activities that make you happy, self-reflection, and connection. A key element of general flourishing is emotional well-being.

Appreciate the Process Rather Than the End Goal:

The beauty of your distinct and growing journey is found in the experiences you've had along the road. Accept the process, draw lessons from setbacks, and savour the opportunities for development.

Avoid Overanalyzing Your Health

Being aware of and making time for your health is crucial, but it's also critical to avoid overanalyzing. A source of empowerment rather than stress should arise from the pursuit of good health. Let the concepts of nourishment become less burdensome and more intuitive by trusting your body and enjoying the trip.

May your life serve as a monument to the possibility for flourishing that each deliberate decision holds, as you carry the wisdom of this all-encompassing book with you. Cheers to a life in which every bite, every conscious instant, every stride is a shining testament to your desire to thrive off the plate. I'm toasting to your pursuit of a lifetime of wellbeing!